Fluid and Electrolytes

24 Hours or Less to Absolutely Crush the NCLEX Exam!

Chase Hassen

Nurse Superhero

© 2015

Disclaimer:

Although the author and publisher have made every effort to ensure that the information in this book was correct at press time, the author and publisher do not assume and hereby disclaim any liability to any party for any loss, damage, or disruption caused by errors or omissions, whether such errors or omissions result from negligence, accident, or any other cause.

This book is not intended as a substitute for the medical advice of physicians. The reader should regularly consult a physician in matters relating to his/her health and particularly with respect to any symptoms that may require diagnosis or medical attention.

NCLEX®, NCLEX®-RN, and NCLEX®-PN are registered trademarks of the National Council of State Boards of Nursing, Inc. They hold no affiliation with this product.

Table of Contents

Have you seen my other NCLEX Prep Books?

NCLEX: Respiratory System : 105 Nursing Practice Questions and Rationales to Easily Crush the NCLEX!

NCLEX: Endocrine System : 105 Nursing Practice Questions and Rationales to EASILY Crush the NCLEX!

NCLEX: Cardiovascular System : 105 Nursing Practice and Rationales to Easily Crush the NCLEX!

NCLEX: Emergency Nursing : 105 Practice Questions and Rationales to Easily Crush the NCLEX!

EKG Interpretation: 24 Hours or Less to Easily Pass the ECG Portion of the NCLEX!

Lab Values: 137 Values You Know to Easily Pass The NCLEX!

First, I want to give you this FREE gift...

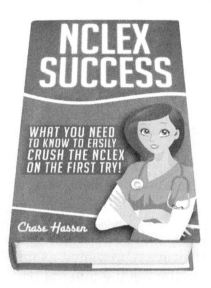

Just to say thanks for downloading my book, I wanted to give you another resource to help you absolutely crush the NCLEX Exam.

For a limited time you can download this book for FREE.

http://bit.ly/1VNGAZ9

Chapter 1:
Introduction

Fluid and electrolyte balance is a very important part of what the body needs to do in order to stay healthy. Fluid is a necessary part of every organ and cell, and fluid makes up much of the extracellular milieu, especially in the blood stream and interstitial fluid (the fluid outside of the cells but not in the bloodstream). Electrolytes represent the mineral content of the bodily fluid. The minerals are in their ionized form, meaning they are represented as mineral ions with an electric charge that makes the mineral part of a salt, acid or base within the body.

For example, sodium and chloride are charged as being positive and negative, respectively. They therefore have a great affinity for one another. When sodium levels are high, for example, there will be a corresponding elevation in chloride. Potassium and chloride are commonly found together within the cells but not so much outside of the cells.

To make matters interesting, there is a great difference in the concentration of electrolytes when comparing the content of electrolytes in the cells as opposed to out of the cells. This difference is maintained by tiny pumps which constantly and instantaneously react to changes in electrolytes within the cells, pumping in potassium and pumping out sodium and their corresponding negatively charged ion. Water balance within the cells is balanced purely by passive movement across the cell membrane.

Which mineral ions are where in the body? The main intracellular ions (charged electrolytes) include potassium, magnesium, phosphorus and sulfate, represented as K+, Mg$_{2+}$, HPO$_2$- and SO$_4$-, respectively. On the other hand, extracellular ions are primarily sodium, calcium, magnesium, chloride and bicarbonate, represented as Na+, Ca$_{2+}$, Mg$_{2+}$, Cl- and HCO3-, respectively. These ions not only are attracted to each other (positive ions are attracted to negative ions) but they are attracted to any charged molecule in the system, making for electrochemically neutral environment both inside and outside the cells.

Besides their function as salts in the body, electrolytes can also make up parts of the acids and bases within the cells and body tissues. Acid-base neutrality with a pH of about 7.4 is necessary within the body for the proper environment for cellular and extracellular enzymatic processes so that, if the electrolytes are not at their proper concentration and the pH level fails to remain at optimal, the enzymatic activity of various body enzymes can be severely compromised.

Humans, as well as nearly all animal forms, require that even subtle changes in electrolytes must be adjusted so as to keep the proper amounts of the various electrolyte salts within the body. These adjustments are particularly important for proper muscle function and nerve function.

Muscle function and the nerves of the body depend on a specific body pH in order to function. This pH balance is maintained by the salts (electrolyte salts) of the body. If the pH is too low or too high, these bodily functions don't work properly. For an example, consider muscle contractions. In order for muscles to contract properly, there must be sufficient amounts of calcium ions, potassium ions and sodium ions. If these are not in their proper concentration, one can develop muscle weakness or an excess of muscle contraction (tetany). Situations of electrolyte imbalance can be life threatening. For this reason, electrolyte imbalances are treated using oral or IV methods.

If a person suffers from an electrolyte imbalance, it can mean that some part of the body's regulating mechanism in maintaining the proper levels of electrolytes is not working properly. Hormones that regulate electrolyte balance include antidiuretic hormone, parathyroid hormone, and aldosterone. In this book, we will discuss these regulating hormones and what happens when they are insufficient or found in excess quantities.

In order for electrolytes to be in the proper concentrations in the body, one must neither be over hydrated nor dehydrated. The kidneys are mostly responsible for keeping the body hydrated to a proper degree. In situations of dehydration or over hydration, the concentrations of the various salts are affected and there can be serious neurological complications, muscle disturbances and heart problems. These situations often call for immediate medical emergency treatment in order to restore the proper electrolyte and water balance.

1.Measuring Electrolyte Levels

For all of the available electrolytes, there are blood tests available to check their level. In fact, part of a basic chemistry profile is the measurements of the various electrolytes of the body. This is done using ion-selective electrode technology that can tell the difference between the different electrically-charged ions. Along with the electrolyte content checked on a blood test, the kidney function is also assessed as the kidneys are partly responsible for what the electrolyte concentration is.

Normally, just the sodium and potassium levels are evaluated with the chloride level calculated from the sodium level provided by the machine. An exception to this is when doing arterial blood gases, in which the chloride level is measured directly along with the blood gas interpretation.

A urine test can also be assessed to see if the electrolytes are properly balanced. When a specific gravity test is done on a urine sample, it can tell if there is an electrolyte imbalance occurring.

When Rehydration is Necessary

In situations of low water content of the body, this usually occurs along with a loss of sodium and potassium, which are excreted in sweat and by the kidneys. If IV supplementation is necessary, it is usually done by hanging a bag of normal saline (which has the proper amount of sodium chloride in the solution and infusing it directly into a peripheral vein. Often potassium is added to the bag of normal saline to make a balanced salt solution for the bloodstream.

Rehydration can also be done orally, if the individual can take in fluids. Water containing sugar for fuel and electrolytes such as is found in oral rehydration solutions like PowerAde and Gatorade can help rehydrate the individual quickly and effectively. Electrolytes can also be given in the form of coconut water, nuts, milk, and fruit juices. Many vegetables and fruits contain electrolytes, whether they be taken whole placed in a juicer. Along with the electrolyte- containing foods, you should drink plenty of water in order to add water to the system.

Dehydration appropriate for oral intake can be a result of exercising too much, sweating in the heat, or even drinking too much alcohol, which acts as a diuretic, resulting in a negative water balance. Each of these conditions lends itself to oral rehydration as long as the individual is conscious and has normal swallowing reflexes.

In this book, we will look at the various electrolytes in the body and find out how they are regulated. We will look at what happens when the different electrolytes are out of balance and will study the purposes of the different electrolytes.

Chapter 2:
Water Balance in the Body

Our body contains more water in it than you might expect. It is estimated that more than half of all our weight is strictly in the form of water. Women have a lesser water percentage than men (55 percent when compared to men at 60 percent. This is because women have more fat in proportion to other body tissues and because fat cells have a lesser percentage of water in them when compared to other types of cells. Children contain more water by percentage at 70 percent when compared to adults; older adults have a lower percentage of body water than younger adults. On average, a 150 pound male has about 10 gallons of water in his system, of which 2/3 to 3/4 is in the cells, with the rest as part of the interstitial fluid (at 7 gallons) or as blood (about one gallon). Water can shift rapidly from one fluid space to another through the process of osmosis.

Because our kidneys constantly excrete water, we must make up for the losses by drinking water in any form. Without proper water intake, the kidneys eventually shut down, we get dehydrated, and we run the risk of electrolyte disturbances that can cause further disarray when it comes to bodily functions. It is better to drink too much water than to drink too little; our kidneys get rid of excess water quite readily as long as they are functioning properly.

Gains and Losses of Water

Water is taken in primarily by drinking water-containing foods. The water is absorbed from the gastrointestinal tract into the bloodstream, where it is distributed where it is needed. Much smaller amounts of water are byproducts of cellular metabolism. This amount of water usually remains in the cell in which the metabolism occurred.

Water is lost by the body in several different ways. The primary way we lose water is through the kidneys, which can filter and excrete many gallons of water in the urine each day, if necessary. Water is also lost through skin evaporation—about 1.5 pints per day. More is lost if we are sweating in the heat. Water is also more humidified going out of the lungs when compared to water taken in through the air, so we lose a small amount of water just in the act of breathing.

Some water is lost through the stool but this varies from person to person. Severe diarrhea can actually result in dehydration as there is not a normal mechanism to conserve water in the GI tract when an inflammatory process in the gut results in water rushing through the GI tract from the blood and into the stool. Vomiting excessively can lead to dehydration as well as diarrhea. Dehydration requires oral or IV water replacement, preferably before the dehydration becomes too severe. If the dehydration comes in the form of excessive vomiting, fluids must be given by IV so that they stay in the system.

Signs and Symptoms of Dehydration

If you become dehydrated for whatever reason, these are the signs and symptoms you might expect to have:

- An increase in thirst
- Feeling sleepy or tired
- Having a dry mouth
- Feeling dizzy
- Having a low urine output with dark yellow urine
- Having no tears when crying
- Having a headache
- Having extremely dry skin with increased "tenting" of the skin when the skin of the back of the hand is pinched
- If you are impaired as to your level of consciousness, you may not feel thirsty and this can impact your ability to take in enough water; instead, IV hydration may be necessary.
- Severe dehydration has additional symptoms than those listed above. A severely dehydrated patient may have:
- A severe lack of urine output of deeply-colored urine
- Rapid heart rate
- A drop in blood pressure when standing (also called orthostatic hypotension)
- Dizziness that is worse upon standing
- Confusion, lethargy or coma
- Fever
- Low skin elasticity
- Seizures
- Shock

These symptoms require immediate IV hydration so as to save the person from dying of their dehydration.

2.Electrolytes in the Body Water

The water in the body has many different substances in it, particularly electrolytes in the form of sodium salts. There is a strong connection between the balance of water and the balance of electrolytes in the body. Because the electrolyte balance is a greater priority, the body will adjust itself as much as is possible to keep the electrolyte concentration the same. If for example, you have an elevation in sodium in the bloodstream, you will experience a desire to drink water in order to dilute out the over-saturated blood stream. The kidneys will also hold onto water so the sodium concentration can be improved.

There is a brain hormone located in the pituitary gland known as vasopressin or antidiuretic hormone (ADH) that is secreted whenever the body senses it is dehydrated. The elevated ADH level will trigger the kidneys to hold onto more water. As you become more hydrated ADH levels fall back down. On the other hand, if the sodium content of the blood is too low, the kidneys are signaled by low levels of ADH to excrete additional water so that the sodium electrolyte balance is restored.

3.Balancing Water in the System

Water is one of the few body molecules that moves passively through osmosis to all areas and compartments of the body. This means that if a cell or body tissue is low in water, the gradient of water is off and water will naturally flow from one area of the body to the needed area. Because the sodium and other electrolyte content of the bloodstream needs to be controlled above all things, there is a natural tendency for blood to passively flow from the cells and interstitial tissue into the bloodstream to maintain normal electrolyte levels.

Chapter 3:
Introduction to Electrolytes

As mentioned, electrolytes are mineral salts that are ionized to form salt, acids and bases in the body. Electrolytes are important in creating the optimum acid-base balance in the body so that enzymes, which have a narrow acceptable pH range, get a chance to continue doing their job. It also means that electrolytes help control the flow of fluid into and out of the cells and various body tissues. When you become dehydrated, for example, it is the elevation in sodium content in the bloodstream that triggers the pituitary gland to secrete more ADH to decrease urine output by the kidneys.

Electrolytes are charged particles of minerals not usually found in their natural non-ionized state in real life. As ions (charged particles), electrolytes have a natural affinity for oppositely charged particles in the system. Sodium can connect with chloride or bicarbonate in the body, depending on need. Electrolytes do not naturally occur ionized without some sort of matching, oppositely charged electrolyte attached to it.

Electrolytes play an important role in cellular metabolism and help the cells maintain cell membrane stability. The body would not function at all without electrolytes, which are found in every fluid space in the body. Sodium chloride is the most common electrolyte salt outside of the cells, whereas potassium chloride is the most common electrolyte within cells. Your body needs this gradient of electrolytes in order to help muscles contract and to help nerve cells generate the electrochemical "current" required to pass impulses from one nerve cell to another. Almost all cellular and extracellular activities in the body are dependent on a certain concentration of salts (electrolytes).

As mentioned, the concentration of sodium, potassium and chloride in the bloodstream need to be critically managed. There are sensors within the kidneys that secrete the hormone renin that helps to keep the electrolyte content of the body within normal limits. Other important hormones in the management of electrolyte content are aldosterone (secreted by the adrenal gland), angiotensin (secreted by the brain, lung and heart tissues), and ADH (secreted by the pituitary gland).

4.The Renin-Angiotensin System

This is a system that operates in order to restore blood pressure when it drops due to any reason, including dehydration or sudden blood loss. When the blood pressure drops, cells in the kidneys secrete the hormone renin in order to restore blood pressure to normal values. Renin attaches to angiotensinogen (which is a hormone secreted by the liver) to form a molecule called angiotensin

- This increases the blood pressure of the system by constricting blood vessels, allowing for an increase in blood pressure. There are medications available for people who have high blood pressure called ACE inhibitors or angiotensin-converting enzyme inhibitors. They block the formation of another molecule called angiotensin II which is the end-point of this system. There are also angiotensin II inhibitors made by pharmaceutical companies that also help to reduce blood pressure by blocking the direct activity of angiotensin II on the blood vessels. Angiotensin-converting enzyme (ACE) is secreted by the lungs.

5.The Function of Aldosterone

Aldosterone is also secreted by the adrenal glands when the person's blood pressure is too low. It causes the kidneys to secrete less water, also raising the blood pressure. It also regulates sodium reuptake in the kidneys so that, if sodium is low, it can decrease the amount of sodium lost by the kidneys and can increase sodium levels in the body. Indirectly it also regulates the hydrogen and potassium levels in the body, effectively regulating the blood pH.

Chapter 4:
Sodium

Sodium is a mineral salt found in high concentrations in the bloodstream and in the interstitial fluid. It is used to keep water in these areas through osmosis and is important in the functioning of the muscles and nerves of the body.

About 85 percent of all body sodium is found in the lymph fluid and blood. Lesser concentrations of sodium are found within the cells. The levels of sodium in the bloodstream are tightly controlled by a aldosterone, a hormone secreted by the adrenal glands. When the sodium level gets low, aldosterone send a signal to the kidneys that tell it to conserve sodium so it isn't lost in the urine. Another source of sodium loss is through sweating; however, this is not controlled and is not a large amount of loss when compared to the kidneys.

We get sodium through our food as sodium in the form of sodium chloride is added to a lot of cooked and premade foods you eat. You can also get sodium in the form of sodium bicarbonate, which is commonly known as baking soda. Medications contain sodium in them, such as toothpaste, mouthwash, laxatives and aspirin.

Sodium in the bloodstream is often paired with chloride to make the common salt, sodium chloride; however, it can be paired with any positively charged molecule including bicarbonate. Because sodium levels need to be tightly regulated, routine blood tests often contain a test for the amount of sodium and chloride in the blood.

A simple, non-fasting blood test can be done in order to determine the level of sodium in the bloodstream. The normal sodium level is about 135-145 mEq/ l, although the actual normal range can vary from testing instrument to testing instrument. When getting your sodium level, check the reference range listed along with your value.

6.Hypernatremia

Hypernatremia is the medical term for high sodium levels. Usually this is not caused by having too much sodium in the body but rather from a loss of water in the body. The main cause of hypernatremia is dehydration where more water than salt is lost from the body so that the relative concentration of sodium is higher than normal.

You can lose water through sweating, diarrhea, urine, and through the expiration of humidified air from the lungs. You can also rarely get hypernatremia through an excessive intake of salt such as when you consume sea water or large amounts of sodium in the diet. For example, eating a lot of soy sauce can contribute to getting too much sodium in the body. This is uncommon, however.

When you experience a rise in sodium concentration in the bloodstream, it triggers the thirst response and you will feel an inordinate need to take in free water. The addition of free water from the gastrointestinal tract will allow for a lowering of the sodium content to normal levels. Hypernatremia is more common in infants, the elderly and those who lack the mental status to drink water or to recognize the need to drink water. Infants and those who suffer from a mental impairment such as Alzheimer's disease generally lack an intact mechanism to recognize that thirst has occurred or cannot get water into their bodies on their own.

7.Signs and Symptoms of Hypernatremia

High sodium levels can cause symptoms, some of which are not very obvious. When you suffer from hypernatremia, you can experience the following symptoms:

1. Weakness

2. Irritability

3. Lethargy

4. Swelling of the tissues

5. Excitability of the nerves and muscles

6. Seizures

7. Coma, often referred to as a hyperosmolar coma

Symptoms can occur with mild elevations of the sodium level, with severe symptoms occurring when the level of sodium reaches 155 mEq/L or more. When the sodium level reaches 180 mEq/ L or greater, the mortality rate is generally quite high, not necessarily from the absolute value of the sodium concentration but because of the underlying and coexisting conditions related to having high sodium concentrations.

8.Causes of Hypernatremia

You can get hypernatremia from a variety of medical causes, including:

- Low intake of enough water to balance the sodium concentration. This is more common in the disabled or elderly population who cannot get free water for themselves due to their disability or to a loss of the thirst response.

- A loss of sodium in the urine that commonly is associated with elevated glucose concentrations. The kidneys must get rid of the glucose and water must go along with that. Sodium stays behind, resulting in a higher concentration of sodium in the bloodstream.

- Extreme sweating results in more water loss than sodium, so you end up with a higher concentration of sodium in the bloodstream.

- Extreme levels of diarrhea which results in more water loss than sodium. The sodium level will be higher in this situation.

- Diabetes insipidus. This is a condition where the body makes little vasopressin in the pituitary gland or when the kidneys do not normally respond to the vasopressin secreted by the pituitary gland.

- Intake of hyperosmolar water. This can be caused when a person takes on too much seawater or receives too much sodium bicarbonate while being resuscitated from a cardiovascular arrest. Seawater contains more sodium in it than the human body so it should not be consumed, even if you are thirsty.

- Salt poisoning. Sometimes young children ingest too much salt so that they will become hypernatremic.

- A rare condition called Conn's syndrome. These people have too much aldosterone in their system and, when faced with a restriction of free water, tend to become hypernatremic.

- Diuretics tend to cause a relatively greater loss of water when compared to sodium so sodium levels increase in the bloodstream.

9.Treatment of Hypernatremia

When a person develops hypernatremia, the treatment of choice is oral or IV free water. Rarely is this given just as free water (when given by IV) but must be given in the form of a dilute solution of dextrose sugar or half normal saline. It is important not to rapidly correct the state of hypernatremia because this can result in rapid shifts of sodium and water within the cells and interstitial fluid so the sodium level must be slowly returned to normal. Water can flow into brain cells when the hypernatremia is fixed too fast, resulting in swelling of the brain and the chance of getting seizures or permanent damage to the brain. The correction of hypernatremia must be done slowly with frequent sodium concentration measurements as the process is happening.

10. Causes of Hyponatremia (Low Sodium)

Low sodium values occur because of excessive sweating, in which you lose sodium as part of salty sweat. If you have severe burns, these will cause fluid loss through the burned skin; an excess of sodium can be lost when compared to water so the sodium levels become low. Poor nutrition is a more rare cause of hyponatremia. There is a medical/psychiatric illness called polydipsia, in which a person drinks excessive amounts of water, diluting out the blood and interstitial fluid.

More uncommon causes of hyponatremia include the following underlying diseases:

- Adrenal failure
- Thyroid gland dysfunction (low thyroid conditions)
- Kidney failure
- Cystic fibrosis
- Liver cirrhosis
- SIADH, which is a syndrome of inappropriate secretion of the hormone, ADH

The treatment of low sodium is to gradually replace the sodium intake, orally or by IV. Like hypernatremia, the treatment of hyponatremia by IV needs to be done slowly so that the sodium and fluid shifts don't adversely affect the cells of the body, particularly the brain.

Sudden changes in sodium level result in more severe and noticeable symptoms when compared to changing sodium levels gradually. Sudden changes in sodium level can result in poor energy levels, confusion, seizures or death.

In order to find out if the kidneys are participating in having too much sodium or too little sodium in the bloodstream, a test is done of the creatinine level of the blood and the urine. These two levels are compared. If there is sodium being excreted in the urine in amounts not appropriate for either low or high sodium in the bloodstream, kidney failure needs to be considered as part of the reason the person has abnormal sodium levels.

Chapter 5:
Chloride

Chloride is the main negative ion in the body, both in the cells and out of the cells. The rise and fall of chloride closely mimics the rise and fall of sodium as they often are found together in an ionic bond within the body tissues. Chloride, in fact, makes up about 70 percent of the normal body negative ions. Chloride makes up about 0.15 percent of the human total body weight, or about 115 grams of chloride. Every day, we take in close to 900 milligrams of chloride per day.

Chloride is one of the major electrolyte ions in the body, found in all areas of the body, paired with either sodium (outside of the cells) or potassium (within the cells). Chloride is responsible, along with the positive ions Na+ and K+, for the electrical messaging between cells, primarily the muscle cells and nerve cells.

11.What does chloride do in the body?

Chloride helps maintain proper osmolality in the body. It also combines with the hydrogen iron in order to make hydrochloric acid, which is a major factor in digestion in the stomach. Hydrochloric acid breaks down ingested proteins, activates intrinsic factor in the stomach, responsible for the body's uptake of vitamin B12. It is transported via chloride channels in the stomach in exchange for bicarbonate, which is another negatively charged ion, in order to create the gradient between hydrochloric acid and sodium hydrochloride outside of the stomach.

Chloride also helps to maintain the pH balance of the bloodstream by actively and passively passing through the red blood cells in exchange for hydrochloride ions so that the body can maintain a pH balance in the bloodstream of around 7.4. In addition, it aids in the release of CO_2 in the respiratory system and helps support the electrical activity that allows for messages to travel from one nerve cell to another or from one muscle cell to another muscle cell. You can't have an excess of ions, positive or negative, in the body, so chloride acts as the primary mineral element within the interstitial fluids, cellular fluids, and the bloodstream.

12. Low Chloride Levels

It is rare to have a chloride deficiency in the body and, when it is low, it usually goes along with a deficiency of sodium as well. Low chloride levels can lead to alkalization of the bloodstream, in which the pH rises above 7.4. This can be life threatening because many enzymes and bodily processes are very dependent upon the pH of the environment and when they don't function well, the body suffers. A common cause of alkalosis of the bloodstream is when one has excessive sodium and chloride ions lost as sodium chloride in the sweat or whenever there is extensive fluid volume loss during prolonged diarrhea and/or vomiting.

Decreased causes of low chloride concentration include:

1. Addison's disease

2. SIADH (syndrome of inappropriate ADH secretion)

3. Metabolic alkalosis

4. Persistent vomiting

5.Congestive heart failure

Symptoms of hypochloremia or low chloride content in the body include irritability leading to lethargy, loss of appetite and dehydration. You can get hypochloremia in much the same way as losses of sodium are incurred—mainly through serious burn injuries, diseases of water overload and starvation, with wasting of the body tissues. Infants can develop hypochloremia if they drink formula that does not contain enough chloride in it. This can cause the infant to fail to thrive, have weakness and exhibit anorexia.

13.High Chloride Levels

It is possible to have high chloride levels in the body, especially when one consumes large amounts of either sodium chloride (table salt) or potassium chloride (salt substitute). Signs and symptoms of an elevated chloride level include high blood pressure and edema (fluid retention). Fortunately, this is a rare condition as the kidneys are usually able to excrete any excess chloride along with sodium or potassium in the form of NaCl or KCl. Another cause of chloride toxicity is congestive heart failure, which can be from disordered metabolism of sodium chloride. Certain kidney diseases hang on to too much chloride, causing hyperchloremia. Most people do not develop a very high level of chloride because their kidneys can excrete any excess chloride in the system, balancing the sodium levels at the same time

Common causes of high chloride in the body include:

2. Excessive salt intake

3. Renal disease

4. Dehydration (such as is seen in vomiting and diarrhea

5. Hyperparathyroidism (an overactive parathyroid gland)

14. Where do we get chloride?

Chloride is found as a part of sodium chloride or table salt. Whenever we consume salty foods, we are causing a relative increase in both sodium and chloride in the blood and interstitial fluids. If you take a salt substitute, such as potassium chloride, you get a matching rise in both potassium and chloride. In this form, the potassium chloride or KCl is mainly found within the cells of the body.

Other sources of chloride include the following:

· Olives

· Rye flour

· Kelp

· Lettuce

· Tomatoes

· Celery

There is a lot of chloride in seawater; however it is not recommended for consumption as the sodium chloride level in sea water is much too high to drink and it can cause both hypernatremia and hyperchloremia. Chloride does not have to be taken as a supplement as it can be found in most foods we eat on a daily basis, unless you consume a very low salt diet. In such cases, chloride would be supplemented with potassium chloride, which is the main salt substitute found on the market.

15.Testing for Chloride in the blood and Urine

Because chloride is such an essential part of health and living, it is often measured as part of an electrolyte profile, a common blood test performed on the body. A urine test can measure the amount of chloride leaving the body through kidney filtration. In order to do this test, all of the urine excreted during a twenty-four hour period of time is collected and the sodium chloride content of the urine is assessed. The levels of potassium, bicarbonate, sodium, and chloride are usually measured from the bloodstream at the same time in order to get an idea of the electrolyte milieu of the body's bloodstream. Chloride can be measured in a special test called the skin sweat test, in which a patch is placed on the arm for a period of time and the electrolytes in the sweat on the patch are measured. This is a test for cystic fibrosis.

16.Normal Values of Chloride in the Body

The normal reference range for chloride varies with age. For example, a normal chloride content in adult blood is 96-106 mEq/L, while newborn infants can have a chloride content in their blood plasma of between 96 and 113 mEq/L. Adults secrete about 140-250 mEq per 24 hour sample in the urine per 24 hours if they have healthy kidney function. Children and toddlers excrete lesser amounts of chloride in the urine, in the range of 15-176 mEq/24 hour sample.

Remember that chloride concentrations go along directly with the levels of sodium and potassium levels as they are found in dissolved form of NaCl and KCl in the body. For this reason, tests of chloride are rarely done alone but are performed in conjunction with the potassium, sodium, and bicarbonate levels of the blood in a chemistry profile. More information can be retrieved from an entire electrolyte panel than can be done by doing electrolyte levels separate from one another.

Chapter 6:
Potassium

Potassium is a necessary mineral and is very important ion in the body. Potassium is of the class of mineral ions, along with sodium, magnesium, calcium, bicarbonate and chloride; it is essential for life in the human body as well as other animals.

Potassium plays a role in the function of skeletal and smooth muscle, including that of the heart and digestive system. As an electrolyte, it conducts electricity, crucial to intercellular communication.

About 98 percent of all potassium is found within the cells. A proper balance of potassium in the cells and sodium outside of the cells is made possible by pumps within the cellular membranes that exchange sodium and potassium, keeping more potassium in the cells.

High potassium is known as hyperkalemia, while low potassium is called hypokalemia. A simple blood test can determine the level of potassium in the blood plasma. Rarely is the potassium checked alone because more information about the electrolyte content of the blood by testing potassium along with sodium, chloride and CO_2 levels together.

17.Uses of Potassium in the Body

The body needs potassium for the function of every cell in the body. These are main functions of potassium:

- Potassium is important in heartbeat regularity

- Potassium levels help determine the blood pressure

- Potassium is important in muscle contraction, including skeletal and smooth muscles Potassium balance is largely controlled by the kidneys, which remove excess potassium through the urine. A normal level of potassium in plasma (the liquid part of blood) is about 3.5 to 5.0 mEq/L. Notice how small this number is when compared to sodium levels, which are high in the bloodstream and low in the cells. The reverse is true with potassium.

18.Causes of Hypokalemia

Hypokalemia is a common problem. It is estimated that nearly one in five persons hospitalized in the US has a potassium level lower than 3.5 mEq/L. The main causes of low potassium include the following conditions:

- Bulimia

- Anorexia nervosa

- The use of diuretic medications

- Bariatric surgery

- Alcoholism

- AIDS patients

- Diarrhea

- Laxative abuse

- Acute or chronic kidney failure
- Low magnesium levels
- Cushing's syndrome
- Leukemia
- Vomiting
- Following an ileostomy
- Steroid use
- Theophylline use
- Overuse of bronchodilators in asthma management
- Taking loop diuretics like Lasix and Bumex
- Taking antacids excessively
- Taking Diflucan for fungal infections

It should be noted that low potassium can increase your chances of getting digoxin toxicity. Digoxin is used to treat heart failure and, while it doesn't cause low potassium levels, low levels of potassium can increase the risk of digoxin toxicity. Potassium levels are often checked in people taking digoxin for that very reason.

19.Symptoms of Hypokalemia

Hypokalemia can be a silent disease, with no or few symptoms. Some symptoms of low potassium include:

- Tingling and/or numbness of the extremities
- Leg or arm muscle cramping
- Fatigue and weakness
- Nausea and/or vomiting
- Constipation
- Extreme thirst along with an increase in urination
- Low blood pressure

- Fainting
- Psychiatric disturbances, such as delirium, psychosis, hallucinations, and confusion
- Heart palpitations

20.Treatment of Hypokalemia

When treating yourself for low potassium levels, you need to avoid any type of heavy physical activity because potassium is lost from the body during sweating. Avoid the use of diuretics, laxatives and any herbal substances that are known to cause hypokalemia. If you suspect you have potassium deficiency, seek a doctor's advice to see what your potassium level is and to get advice or medication to control the potassium level in the body.

Potassium levels can be brought up by using intravenous or oral medications. Care must be taken when increasing the potassium levels by IV means because it is easy to overshoot the target and cause hyperkalemia. Hyperkalemia can cause severe heart beat abnormalities so that anyone getting potassium replaced needs to be placed on a cardiac monitor which can tell if an abnormal beat has occurred. IV replacement of potassium should be reserved for potassium levels less than mEq/L. Returning the potassium level to normal levels needs to be done as slowly as possible to allow for shifts in potassium and water levels within and outside of the cells and so as to prevent heart problems associated with having a high potassium levels.

When a doctor prescribes oral potassium replacement for low potassium levels, the potassium should be rechecked every two to three days until the potassium levels normalize. If the cause of the hypokalemia is due to the use of a diuretic, you may need to switch to a potassium-sparing diuretic or combine a potassium-sparing diuretic with a potassium-losing diuretic for high blood pressure or fluid retention.

21.Preventing Low Potassium Conditions

If you are at risk for low potassium, there are good food sources of potassium, particularly in the following fruits, meats and vegetables:

· Tomatoes

· Cantaloupes

· Bananas

· Oranges

· Peaches

· Potatoes

· Avocados

· Flounder

· Lima beans

· Chicken

· Cod or salmon

If you are at risk for hypokalemia, you should have your potassium checked every 3-6 months and sooner if you have symptoms of low potassium.

22.Hyperkalemia

In some ways, hyperkalemia or "high potassium" is more dangerous than hypokalemia because high levels of potassium can cause heart arrhythmias and sudden death. The main causes of hyperkalemia include the use of potassium-sparing diuretics and kidney failure. If your kidneys are not working, potassium will not be properly excreted and the potassium level will rise. Addison's disease, in which low levels of aldosterone are in the system, the potassium level will rise to above normal levels.

- There are many different medications that can cause elevated potassium levels. Consider these as possible causes if a patient has high potassium levels and are on any of these medications:

- Antibiotics, like trimethoprim or penicillin

- ACE inhibitors for high blood pressure

- Medications for yeast infections, particularly the azole type medications

- Heparin, for thinning the blood

- NSAIDS, for fever and pain from inflammation

- Herbal supplements such as Siberian ginseng, milkweed, Hawthorn berries, lily of the valley and ground toad skin preparations

- Supplements containing potassium

- Potassium-sparing diuretics, including spironolactone and triamterene

23.Symptoms of Hyperkalemia

The major symptoms of hyperkalemia include the possibility of life threatening heart arrhythmias, bradycardia (slow heart rate) and muscle weakness. If the potassium level is not yet dangerously high, you may have no symptoms at all. A simple lab test can confirm the diagnosis of hyperkalemia. As always, potassium levels are best interpreted in light of checking other electrolytes at the same time. An EKG can show changes consistent with markedly elevated levels of potassium in the bloodstream.

24.Treatment of High Potassium Levels

If the potassium level is extremely high, you need to consider medication that helps reduce the total body amount of potassium. These include the following:

- Diuretics that promote potassium loss in the urine
- IV glucose and insulin, which fills the cells with potassium as well
- Sodium polystyrene sulfonate, which gets rid of potassium through the GI tract
- Kidney dialysis
- Calcium infusion by IV to correct heart rhythm abnormalities

25.Benefits of Potassium

Diets high in potassium have been found to improve bone density among older women. People who are deficient in potassium seem to have higher blood pressure than those who have enough potassium in their system. Potassium in the diet is related to stroke prevention. People with Crohn's disease or ulcerative colitis don't absorb potassium as well as normal people so that they often need potassium supplementation.

26.Taking Potassium supplements

You should always talk to your doctor to see if you need potassium supplementation. There are side effects to taking potassium, such as irritation of the stomach, abnormal heart rate and diarrhea. If you take enough potassium to cause high potassium levels (for example, you should not take potassium supplements if you have kidney failure) you can develop muscle weakness, abnormal rhythms of the heart or bradycardia (slow heart beat). Those who take ACE inhibitors, Bactrim, Septra, or potassium-sparing diuretics, should not take potassium supplementation. The same is true for those who take NSAIDs for inflammation or pain. Beta blocker medication can raise potassium levels.

Chapter 7:
Magnesium

Magnesium is actually a common mineral in the body; it is used frequently as a cofactor in more than 300 cellular reactions within the cells. Magnesium is important in energy production, glycolysis, blood sugar control, protein synthesis, muscle function, blood pressure regulation and nerve production. Magnesium is essential for bone health and is an essential cofactor in DNA and RNA synthesis. Magnesium is necessary to run the pumps involved in the transportation of potassium ions and calcium ions into and out of the cells. This is extremely necessary in muscle contraction, the maintenance of heart rhythm, and the conduction of nerve impulses.

At any given point in time, our body contains about 25 grams of magnesium of which more than fifty percent is found in bone. The rest, around 40-50 percent is found in the soft tissue cells with only one percent residing in serum. The normal range of magnesium in a blood test of serum reveals an average value of 0.75 to 0.95 mmol/L. Any number lower than 0.75 mmol/L is considered hypomagnesemia and any number above 0.95 percent is considered to be hypermagnesemia. The homeostasis of magnesium occurs primarily through proper kidney function, which excretes about 120 mg of magnesium daily. If the magnesium levels are low, the kidneys will hold onto more magnesium in order to achieve homeostasis.

Because the vast majority of magnesium is sequestered in soft tissue and bone, the absolute amount of magnesium is difficult to determine with just a blood test. One of the best tests in assessing the total body levels of magnesium is to give a dose of magnesium by IV and to assess the level of magnesium in the urine after that. If the magnesium content of the urine is low despite receiving a bolus of magnesium, it is likely that there are low levels of magnesium in the body.

The recommended dietary allowances or RDAs for magnesium vary with age. For example, in small infants, the RDA for magnesium is only 30 grams per day, while in adults the RDA is between 310 mg and 420 mg per day. Men require more magnesium than women.

27.Magnesium Sources

Ideally we should get our magnesium through the food we eat, although some people would benefit from magnesium supplementation. Great sources of magnesium are legumes, almonds, spinach and other greens, seeds, whole grains and other nuts. Food high in fiber tends also to be high in magnesium. Certain bottled waters and even tap water can be good sources of magnesium intake. Of the magnesium we take into our bodies, only about 30-40 percent is actually absorbed by the gastrointestinal tract.

You can purchase magnesium supplements in the form of a magnesium salt made as magnesium citrate, magnesium oxide and magnesium chloride. When reading the label, the magnesium amount is the weight of the magnesium alone and not the weight of the magnesium salt in the supplement. Magnesium citrate, magnesium lactate, magnesium chloride and magnesium aspartate are particular magnesium supplements that are readily bioavailable once taken in. High zinc intake can interfere with the absorption of magnesium.

Certain laxatives contain high doses of magnesium such as Phillip's Milk of Magnesia®. Certain heartburn medications also contain a great deal of magnesium. Rolaids® is an example of a high source of magnesium.

28.Low Magnesium Levels

Hypomagnesemia is relatively rare due to the ability of the kidneys to hold onto magnesium in times of low magnesium intake. Chronic alcoholism, on the other hand, represents a state of chronically low magnesium and this is a situation where supplemental magnesium needs to be considered.

Signs and symptoms of magnesium deficiency include nausea and vomiting, fatigue and weakness, and poor appetite. Severe hypomagnesemia can cause paresthesias (tingling and numbness) of the extremities, muscle cramps, abnormal heart rhythms, seizures and changes in personality. When the intake of magnesium is low and the blood levels are low, one will also find similar disruptions of calcium and potassium in the bloodstream.

Risk factors for hypomagnesemia include type 2 diabetics, GI diseases that interfere with mineral absorption, alcoholics, the elderly and those with kidney dysfunction. Low levels of potassium can lead to the development of certain diseases, including high blood pressure, osteoporosis, heart disease, type 2 diabetes, and migraines. Magnesium supplementation seems to decrease the risk of sudden cardiovascular death. Stroke is also decreased in those people who have high magnesium levels and type 2 diabetes risk is directly associated with low magnesium levels in the blood. An intake of about 100 mg of magnesium per day has been found to reduce the incidence of type 2 diabetes by 15 percent.

Magnesium is a necessary part of bone growth, influencing the activities of osteoclasts and osteoblasts. Magnesium content affects the parathyroid gland and the amount of vitamin D in the system—both of which regulate the homeostasis of bone growth and mineral content. Some studies have linked low magnesium levels with an increased risk of osteoporosis.

Magnesium loss or poor intake of magnesium is related to the formation of migraine headaches. While this is true, magnesium supplementation doesn't always treat or reduce the number of migraine headaches a person has. Some researchers recommend magnesium intakes of 600 mg per day in divided doses can prevent frequent migraine headaches.

29.High Magnesium Levels

While you can't really suffer from a high magnesium level when you get magnesium from foods, certain supplements, when taken in excess, can raise magnesium levels above the normal range.

High dose magnesium from medications or supplements can lead to crampy abdominal pain, nausea, vomiting, and diarrhea. The laxative effects of magnesium salts are believed to be due to the osmotic effect of having so much magnesium salt in the colon. High magnesium levels also increase gastric motility. Magnesium toxicity can rarely be fatal, especially among the very young and the very old. The risk of hypermagnesemia is highest in those who suffer from renal dysfunction (kidney failure) so that the kidneys fail to get rid of excess magnesium in the diet.

30.Medication Interactions

Magnesium supplementation strongly affects the efficacy of certain medications. For example, magnesium can interfere with the absorption of medications used to treat osteoporosis, primarily the bisphosphonate-type medications, the absorption of tetracycline, the absorption of quinolone antibiotics, proton pump inhibitors like Nexium® and Prevacid®. Magnesium loss can be found when a person takes diuretics such as Lasix® or hydrochlorothiazide in excess for long periods of time.

31.Dietary Intake of Magnesium

Magnesium can come from eating a healthier diet. For example, magnesium can be taken in when eating a wide variety of fruits and vegetables along with whole grains and milk products. Spinach contains high levels of magnesium and certain breakfast cereals will be supplemented with magnesium. Meat, poultry, eggs, nuts, beans and fish are high in magnesium and make for good magnesium levels in the body. Soybeans and legumes like peanuts, lentils and baked beans are high in magnesium. Whole grains in the form of millet and brown rice contain adequate amounts of magnesium as well.

Chapter 8:
Calcium

Calcium is the most common form of mineral in the body with the vast majority of calcium being in the bones and teeth (99 percent). Calcium is also used for proper functioning of the nerves, the heart, the muscles, and other body symptoms.

Calcium isn't absorbed nor is it used well if not for the concomitant presence of phosphorus, magnesium, vitamin K and vitamin D. While calcium supplements are plentiful, the best source of absorbable calcium is through the food you eat. Calcium intake is especially important among young children who are continually growing bones and teeth, as well as in pregnant women. Calcium supplements are generally reserved for the following groups of people:

- People who use a lot of caffeine
- Heavy alcohol drinkers
- Postmenopausal women
- Soda drinkers
- Those who take corticosteroids

32. Purposes of Calcium in the Body

Calcium plays a large role in bone formation and maintenance. Bone loss accelerates after age thirty so that by the time a person is elderly, osteoporosis is more common.

Bone loss can be prevented by supplementing the diet with calcium and vitamin D. People who have lost their parathyroid glands due to thyroid surgery suffer from low calcium and phosphorus and should take a calcium and vitamin D supplement. They should also refrain from taking in too much phosphorus. Women who suffer from premenstrual syndrome have been found to reduce their symptoms when they take 1,200 mg of calcium per day. This reduces the physical symptoms of PMS, such as bloating, mood disturbances, headache, and food cravings.

Those who suffer from low body calcium levels seem to be at a higher risk of developing high blood pressure. This has been shown in several studies although it is not known if calcium supplementation would turn around high blood pressure on its own. Calcium may prevent high blood pressure in people predisposed to the condition. There have been studies linking high dose calcium intake (up to 2000 mg per day) can reduce their cholesterol levels. Rickets, while rare now, is a disease linked to not getting enough calcium in the diet. People at risk for stroke may benefit from taking a calcium supplement and there is some evidence that calcium along with vitamin D is preventative against colon cancer.

33.Causes of Low Calcium

The most common cause of low calcium is hypoparathyroidism. Everyone has four tiny parathyroid glands imbedded in the thyroid gland. If the thyroid gland has to be removed for any reason and if the parathyroid glands go with it, there can be problems with low calcium and high phosphorus levels.

There is an autoimmune variant of hypoparathyroidism in which antibodies are made against the calcium-sensing receptors in the parathyroid glands. A person can also be born with a congenital defect involving the calcium-sensing receptors. Another hereditary condition causing low calcium is DiGeorge syndrome, in which the parathyroid glands fail to develop.

Low magnesium levels affect the parathyroid hormones and very high magnesium levels lead to an inhibition of parathyroid hormone so that the calcium level may be low. Vitamin D and calcium deficiency combined will result in low calcium levels. Phosphate administration will lower calcium concentrations and acute pancreatitis allows for the deposition of calcium in the abdomen so less calcium is available in the bloodstream. Metastatic cancer (particularly from the breast and prostate gland) will lower the blood calcium levels. Several types of chemotherapy will lower blood calcium levels as well.

34.Signs and Symptoms of Hypocalcemia

If the hypocalcemia is of a gradual onset or is mild, there may be no symptoms at all. If there is a sudden or severe loss of calcium, the patient may suffer from tetany of the muscles and hyperactivity of the nerves. There can be numbness or tingling sensations of the fingertips and around the mouth. People with low calcium levels can suffer from muscle cramps. Breathing can be affected if the muscles required for breathing are in spasm. Other symptoms of low calcium include:

· Dementia or mental retardation

· Seizure activity

· Anxiety or depression

· Parkinson's symptoms

· Brain calcifications

· Increased muscular irritability

· Low blood pressure or heart failure

- Sweating
- Asthma symptoms (bronchospasm)

35.Diagnosing Low Calcium

A person is said to have hypocalcemia if they have a total serum calcium level of less than 8.2 mg/dL or an ionized level lower than 4.4 mg/dL. The physical examination may show some of the signs noted above. Patients who have chronic kidney disease or who lost their parathyroid gland function are all at risk for low calcium concentration in the blood.

36.Treatment of Hypocalcemia

Treatment of hypocalcemia can benefit from IV replacement with calcium gluconate. The first 1-2 grams of calcium gluconate should be given slowly over 10-20 minutes as too rapidly replacing calcium can affect heart rhythm. Calcium can irritate the veins so it should be highly diluted in normal saline or dextrose solutions. Check the magnesium level in all patients with low calcium because the two can go together and magnesium may need to be replaced as well. Replacement should be slow and gradual especially in patients who suffer from kidney damage. Calcium is often given along with vitamin D for maximum effectiveness. Diuretic therapy can also increase the kidneys' abilities to hang onto calcium.

37.Signs and Symptoms of High Calcium Levels

With high calcium levels, there can be overworking of the kidneys, leading to thirstiness and frequent urination. You can get abdominal pain, nausea, vomiting, or constipation from high calcium levels. The excess calcium in the bloodstream usually comes from a leaching of calcium out of the bones, so you can get bony pain and osteoporosis. You can have weakness of the muscles and brain symptoms such as confusion, fatigue and malaise.

38.Calcium Supplementation

The best dietary sources of calcium come from dairy products, including milk, cheeses and yogurt. Blackstrap molasses and tofu are rich in calcium. Certain nuts, cabbage, broccoli, kelp and dark leafy greens contain a great deal of calcium as well. Non-plant sources of calcium include fortified cereals, salmon, oysters and sardines.

You can buy calcium supplements with or without vitamin D. Calcium citrate is the easiest to absorb when compared to calcium carbonate; however, the latter is cheaper to buy. Calcium carbonate should be taken with orange juice or other acidic drink because this helps the calcium to absorb better.

The dose of calcium supplements vary with age. Newborns and infants should receive about 200 mg per day, while adults up to age 50 need 1000 mg per day. Women who are postmenopausal may need up to 1,200 mg of calcium daily.

There are side effects whenever you take calcium supplements. This can include constipation, stomach indigestion, confusion, renal failure, and irregular heartbeats. If you have hyperparathyroidism, cancer, kidney failure or sarcoidosis, you shouldn't take calcium by means of supplementation and should get calcium strictly from the diet.

Calcium supplementation should be taken under the care of your doctor if you are taking bisphosphonates such as Fosamax® or Didronel®. Aluminum containing antacids can cause an elevated absorption of calcium citrate. Blood pressure medications like beta-blockers and calcium channel blockers can be interfered with if you take calcium supplementation.

People on digoxin for heart failure may experience toxicity to digoxin, while low levels of calcium interfere with the activity of digoxin. Thiazide diuretics can raise the calcium level in the bloodstream, while loop diuretics like Lasix® can reduce calcium levels. Calcium supplements can block quinolone antibiotic absorption and tetracycline absorption. Dilantin® and other seizure medication can reduce serum calcium levels.

Chapter 9:
Phosphorus

Phosphorus is the second most common mineral found in the human body, just behind calcium. Phosphorus is essential for proper health; it is used in enzymatic reactions that grow and repair tissues of the body. A total of 85 percent of the phosphorus in the body is found in your bones and teeth, providing strong bones and teeth.

39. Purposes of Phosphorus

The phosphorus molecule is found inside the body as the phosphate ion. Phosphates are essential to making ATP, which is the main energy molecule in the body. The phosphorus in ATP is lost during an energy reaction in which ATP (adenosine triphosphate) turns into ADP (adenosine diphosphate), releasing energy to power cellular reactions.

Phosphorus is also a major component of DNA and RNA in the cells. Without phosphorus, we would have no genetic blueprint within the cells. If we don't get enough phosphorus, protein synthesis is impaired and the cells of the body suffer.

Phosphorus is a natural buffer which acts to neutralize acids in the body so that the pH is kept at 7.4. The hemoglobin in our bloodstream and many bodily enzymes make use of phosphorus as a cofactor or as a part of the structure of the protein itself.

40.Where do you get phosphorus in the diet?

Much of the phosphorus in our diet comes from a wide variety of foods, such as eggs, milk, fish, legumes, grains and cereals. Carbonated beverages of any type contain a lot of phosphorus, even though they are not always healthful in other ways. Food additives also have a great deal of phosphorus in them. It is recommended that we take in about 700 mg of phosphorus daily. Amounts of phosphorus exceeding 4 grams per day are not healthy for you so you should watch your phosphorus intake, especially if you have kidney problems. The calcium intake in your diet should roughly match the amount of phosphorus in your diet because bones and teeth require equal amounts of these minerals. It is rare to have a phosphorus deficiency because it is so plentiful in the diet.

41.Low Phosphorus Levels

Certain medications, such as antacids and diuretics, can cause a reduction in the serum phosphorus content. Other conditions can result in a low phosphorus content, such as type 2 diabetes, alcoholism, and starvation. Diseases of the bowel such as celiac disease and Crohn's disease can be so severe as to limit the amount of phosphorus and other minerals absorbed by the GI tract. In such cases, the phosphorus levels can be too low.

If the phosphorus level is too low, some symptoms can be anxiety, bony pain, lack of appetite, osteoporosis, fatigue, joint stiffness, numbness, irritability, breathing problems and weight fluctuations. Children with low phosphorus levels do not grow properly because they need phosphorus for healthy bone growth and teeth formation.

42.High Phosphorus Content

Too much phosphorus in the bloodstream happens more commonly that low phosphorus situations. High phosphorus can be because of kidney disease, taking too much phosphorus in the diet or consuming too little calcium, which must balance out with the amount of phosphorus you take in. High phosphorus levels are linked to an increase in cardiovascular disease risk. Too much phosphate in your system can lead to phosphorus toxicity, leading to diarrhea and hardening of the arteries (atherosclerosis). Too much phosphate can also lead to an interference with the ability of the body to use calcium, zinc, magnesium and iron. Some athletes take phosphorus before strenuous activity to prevent muscle stiffness. This should only be done under a doctor's care so that the phosphorus level doesn't get too high.

Ideally, there should be a balance between the calcium and phosphorus intake in the body. Unfortunately, modern western diets contain a great deal more phosphorus than calcium and calcium must be leached from bones and teeth in order to match the amount of phosphorus in the bloodstream; the bones can become brittle.

Chapter 10:
Conclusion

It is a serious understatement to say that electrolytes are necessary for life. Electrolytes are charged mineral particles that create the environment of our cells and our interstitial fluid. Sodium and potassium, along with chloride and bicarbonate, set the stage for the environmental milieu and keep the amount of water in the various body compartments as stable as possible.

Minerals ions are used as cofactors in enzymatic reactions that are part of cellular metabolism. They can also be used as part of the enzymes themselves. Phosphorus, for example, is a big part of cellular ATP, used to create the energy needed for cellular functions. Phosphorus also makes up the substance of our nuclear material, such as DNA and the various types of RNA.

Much of the electrolyte balance in our bodies is determined by the kidneys, which filter electrolytes and respond to changes in electrolyte concentration of the blood by holding onto or excreting electrolytes in order to maintain proper electrolyte concentrations in the body. If you suffer from kidney failure, the electrolytes do not balance properly and there can be excesses or deficiencies of certain electrolytes.

Electrolyte balance is a big part of homeostasis in the body. There is, by necessity, more potassium in the cells than in the bloodstream and more sodium in the bloodstream than in the cells. This homeostasis is managed by potassium and sodium pumps that create the marked difference between the intracellular milieu and the extracellular milieu.

Most diets contain enough of the various electrolytes, with the exception of possibly calcium. The intake of phosphorus should ideally keep up with the intake of calcium as they are used in equal quantities in bones and teeth. Unfortunately, Western diets are much too high in phosphorus intake when compared to calcium intake so that calcium is leached from the bone in order to maintain bloodstream concentrations of calcium and phosphorus that are equal to one another. This can lead to brittle bones.

Electrolytes create an environment in which the enzymes can work properly for all the various reactions necessary for health. The cellular and extracellular quantities of the various electrolytes determine the pH of these tissue areas so that enzymatic processes can happen in the proper pH range.

If you enjoyed this book, would you be kind enough to leave a review on Amazon? Your positive reviewers can help others to see what kinds of helpful resources are out there!

Thank you and good luck on your medical endeavors!

- Chase Hassen

Nurse Superhero

Highly Recommended Books for Success

1. NCLEX: Cardiovascular System : 105 Nursing Practice and Rationales to Easily Crush the NCLEX!

2. NCLEX: Emergency Nursing : 105 Practice Questions and Rationales to Easily Crush the NCLEX!

3. Lab Values: 137 Values You Know to Easily Pass The NCLEX!

4. EKG Interpretation: 24 Hours or Less to Easily Pass the ECG Portion of the NCLEX!

5. Fluid and Electrolytes: 24 Hours or Less to Absolutely Crush the NCLEX Exam!

6. Nursing Careers: Easily Choose What Nursing Career Will Make Your 12 Hour Shift a Blast!

7. Night Shift: 10 Survival Tips for Nurses to Get Through The Night!

8. NCLEX: Endocrine System : 105 Nursing Practice Questions and Rationales to EASILY Crush the NCLEX!

And **MUCH MUCH MORE**! Visit my amazon author page to see more at http://amzn.to/1HCtfSy

Made in the USA
Las Vegas, NV
13 October 2023

79047552R00036